Caregiving

Taking Care of Yourself
While Caring for Someone Else

DEBBIE BARR

AspirePress

Caregiving: Taking Care of Yourself
While Caring for Someone Else

Copyright © 2024 Deborah Barr
Published by Aspire Press
An imprint of Tyndale House Ministries
Carol Stream, Illinois
www.hendricksonrose.com

ISBN: 978-1-4964-8351-5

Author photo by Melinda Lamm. Cover photo: Ground Picture/ Shutterstock.com. Other images used under license from Shutterstock.com.

Printed in the United States of America
010923VP

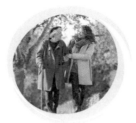

Contents

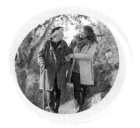

Introduction
The Caregiving Journey

CAREGIVING HAS BEEN DESCRIBED AS A JOURNEY. However, it's not the "traveling-from-one-place-to-another" kind of journey. It's a journey of compassion, walking alongside someone coping with illness or disability or the effects of aging. But caregiving is never just about the person needing care. No matter who you're caring for, or why, or for how long, the caregiving journey is *always also* about you, the caregiver.

Most of the time, caregiving is an *unexpected* journey. Few family caregivers ever foresee the day when a tragic accident, a mental or physical illness, or dementia would put them in a caregiving role. While everyone understands that health often declines with age, few of us are fully prepared to meet the challenges of caring for an elderly loved one. So, whether the caregiving journey is short term or for the long haul, more often than not, it's an unplanned journey into unknown territory. And for so very many, it's not an easy journey.

Caregiving can be exhausting! It's not unusual for caregivers to feel overwhelmed, stressed out, or to even get sick themselves while caring for someone else. For some, it's also a lonely journey, because they don't have enough support or help. And even though it's one of the most important jobs anyone can ever do, caregiving can take a surprising toll on body, mind, and spirit.

But here's the great news: your caregiving experience doesn't have to be like that! When caregiving tasks are shared and caregivers understand how to take care of themselves as well as their family member, the whole experience is much brighter for everyone.

This book will help you create a "best case scenario" caregiving experience for both your loved one and for you. Because caregivers need care too, this book is not as much about care *giving* as about care *receiving*. It's a book about *self-care* for caregivers.

Do you think "self-care" sounds, well ... selfish? Do you wonder if self-care really even matters?

As you will discover on the pages ahead, caregiver self-care does matter—a lot. It's not optional, and it's definitely not selfish. In fact, it's very smart and very necessary. Well-meaning caregivers sometimes sacrifice their own physical, emotional, and other needs so they can pour all their energy and devote all their time to the person in their care. While that sounds noble and loving, it's not. It actually puts the cared-for person at risk.

Does that surprise you? Here's the truth. If you ignore your own needs for restful sleep, healthy food, exercise, medical care, spiritual nurture, and "time off," sooner or later, you will be *unable* to go on meeting the needs of the person in your care. Unless you make caring for yourself a top priority, you may burn out or bail out. And where would that leave the person you're caring for?

Self-care is what will enable you to endure the challenges of caregiving. It keeps your emotional, spiritual, and physical reserves from running out. It equips you to be the patient, loving, and truly *caring* caregiver you want to be.

On the pages ahead, you will hear from my "panel of experts," Jean and Mark, two full-time family caregivers who understand the wisdom and necessity of self-care. Both have found the balance between caring well for their loved ones and caring well for themselves. I say loved *ones,* because each has walked the difficult journey of caring for two people at the same time. While that's twice the work, neither of these caregivers would hesitate to say that it's also twice the blessing.

Maybe you have been a caregiver for a long time, or maybe you have just started your caregiving journey. Either way, you probably have something in common with Jean and Mark, and you will, no doubt, benefit from their wise perspectives on self-care while on the caregiving journey.

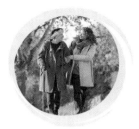

Chapter 1
The Upside and Downside of Caregiving

JEAN AND HER HUSBAND, RYAN, HAVE THREE ADULT children. Two of them, a thirty-three-year-old daughter and a thirty-six-year-old son, are on the autism spectrum. As young children, they displayed few symptoms and family life was fairly normal. At puberty, however, both children changed dramatically. Doctors suspect that hormone changes triggered mitochondrial disease and autism. Since their early teenage years, Jean has cared for both her son and her daughter at home. Recently, her higher-functioning daughter moved into a supervised care residence. Jean now cares full time for her son, Daniel, who is unable to communicate his needs and unable to tend to his own personal daily hygiene.

Mark cares full time for his wife, Michelle, who has Parkinson's disease. In the past year Mark has faced seemingly endless caregiving challenges as Michelle has struggled to recuperate from four surgeries and a serious infection. Though the surgeries and infection were unrelated to Parkinson's, they greatly complicated the care Mark had to provide. At times, he provided round-the-clock care, giving Michelle medicine late at night and early in the morning, robbing him of sleep. For months, Michelle was unable to walk, creating a challenge for Mark to safely take her to doctor's visits. At home, he has needed to bathe Michelle and help her get around in their home. All the while, Mark was also overseeing the medical and financial aspects of his ninety-two-year-old mother's care in an assisted living facility. He continues to do that and must leave Michelle in the care of others when he needs to be with his mom.

Like many family caregivers, Jean and Mark had never envisioned themselves in their caregiving roles. Fortunately, they each had experiences that helped prepare them for what lay ahead. Jean, a registered nurse, had years of experience caring for patients in many different settings. Mark had previously helped care for his mentally ill mother-in-law and for his father who had dementia.

However, not everyone has some training or experience that helps them get comfortable with caregiving. If you do, you may feel somewhat prepared for whatever may lie ahead. But if you're new to caregiving, with no helpful training or experiences to rely on, it's normal to wonder if you're up to the task.

Whether you are a seasoned caregiver or just starting out, it's not uncommon to feel alone and lacking in support from others. If that's how you feel, you might be encouraged to know that there are a great many others traveling the same road as you. About 1 in every 5 Americans is a caregiver—that's about 53 million people! And you're not even alone in feeling alone. About 1 out of 5 caregivers of adults reports feeling alone.[1] Happily, there's a wonderful cure for the aloneness of caregiving. In fact, one goal of this book is to help you surround yourself with a team of supportive people.

And it's very important to have a team now that you're moving to … *France*.

What, you didn't know you were moving to France? Just kidding. You're not *actually* moving to France, of course! "Moving to France" is Jean's way of saying that, for her, caregiving has been like suddenly finding yourself in a foreign country. She says it's like planning to live in England but realizing that "God has you in France." Jean's plan for her life didn't include long-term caregiving. Though she was deeply committed to her children, it was hard to adapt when the severity of both their conditions took her life on a very unexpected detour. She remembers feeling like this:

> You prepare for England. You learn the language of England and you study the customs of England. You're all ready to live in England. And all of a sudden you wake up in France! You don't know the language. You don't know the culture. *"I was supposed to be in England! I planned to be in England—and here I am in France."*

There was no choice about caregiving, of course, and Jean admits, "I wouldn't have picked it." At first, she had more questions than answers and no real clue about which way to turn. But as a loving mom, she forged ahead, telling herself, "Well, you've just got to learn the French way now."

The Upside of Caregiving

Fast forward to the present day. Jean has now been a full-time caregiver for more than twenty years. In the early years, when she felt so lost and overwhelmed, her children's diagnoses were unknown, and her only support was her husband. For a long time, the caregiving journey was extremely difficult. In time, however, Jean found the community resources and the support she was looking for. That much-needed help tremendously lightened her load. Even more importantly, as the years passed, Jean learned to pay more attention to her own needs. To this day, she continues to practice self-care that enables her not just to survive, but to thrive as a long-term caregiver. She describes her life today with words that might surprise you: *rich* and *abundant*. After more than twenty years of caregiving, how is *that* possible?

Attitude Is Everything.

Jean explains, "Caregivers live life on a different level because the job is so consuming. However, it's all about the attitude we choose. Attitude is everything. I do not look at being a caregiver for someone who is mentally or physically ill as a heartbreak. If it is seen as a heartbreak, it will be reflected in everything you do." It is this attitude that also enables Jean to look back through the years and conclude, "My son's disability has blessed us in ways that I would never have guessed."

Mark also believes that "attitude is everything." He says that if care is given with bitterness, "then you're angry, then you're in a bad mood. And then you don't treat anyone else lovingly, including the person that you care for."

A Sense of Purpose

Many family caregivers say that caring for their loved one has given them a sense of purpose and made their lives more meaningful. When I asked Mark if he felt more of a sense of burden or more of a sense of purpose in his caregiving, he responded, "Purpose for sure. It is my joy to care for my wife during this difficult time in her life." Jean's outlook is similar: "It's been hard, but it's been rich and meaningful."

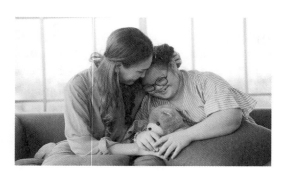

For both Mark and Jean, caregiving has also been spiritually meaningful. Jean reflected, "I didn't realize that praying for a meaningful life meant it would be difficult. But when we're in the valley we really sense God more than when we're on the hilltops." Mark said it gives him peace knowing that "God's got this." A survey conducted by the National Opinion Research Center found that 83 out of 100 caregivers thought of caregiving as a positive experience. Many also reported a sense of satisfaction in caring for someone who had once cared for them or felt satisfaction in providing excellent care for a loved one.[2]

The Caregiving in the United States report found that of the nearly 1,500 caregivers surveyed, more than half said caregiving has given them a sense of purpose or meaning in life.[3] This survey also revealed that:

- Those who had a choice about caregiving felt more of a sense of purpose than those who had no choice.

- More primary (main) caregivers felt a sense of purpose than non-primary caregivers.

- Those providing care in high intensity situations or for many hours per week felt a greater sense of purpose than those providing care for fewer hours or in low intensity situations.

Ponder those survey results for a moment. Do you find it interesting (I do!) that caregivers in the more difficult, more time-consuming situations felt a greater sense of purpose than those in easier circumstances?

The C.A.R.E. study found that:[4]

- 42% of caregivers say they often feel pride for "doing the right thing."

- 37% say they feel that same pride *all the time.*

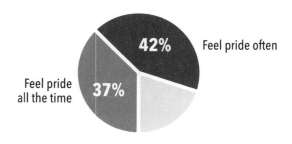

Love the Person.

If you know a family caregiver like Jean or Mark, you may have marveled at their perseverance. You may have even wondered, "How do they *do* this day in and day out? Do they have some special superpower?"

Actually, there *is* something special, and in a sense, a kind of superpower that energizes caregivers and enables them to faithfully keep on keeping on. Not all caregivers have discovered it yet, but it's no secret. In fact, while Mark probably wouldn't call it a superpower, he doesn't hesitate to say that it's the one thing that keeps him motivated to care for Michelle day after day, on good days and especially on not-so-good days.

"To do this," he explained, "*you have to love the person.* Or love the person that person belongs to." Reflecting on his years helping to care for his first wife's mother, he said, "I loved my wife dearly, and that's why I loved her mother."

Mark's experience with his former mother-in-law was not always pleasant and not often predictable. He remembers, "I would have to psych myself up to go see her, because I never knew what I was going to find with her mental illness." Even so, he says, "There was joy in the caregiving. I learned to love her."

Mark's experience with his dad was similar. His dad was an extrovert with a big personality that shone through in spite of his dementia. Mark recalls, "I never knew what was going to come out of his mouth!" But, he says, "There was joy in the caregiving with my dad too. I didn't know how long he had, but I just kept showing up and loving him right where he was."

Now Mark's aging mother and his wife, Michelle, are experiencing that same faithful love from Mark, their mutual caregiver.

It is also this kind of faithful love that motivates Jean to be the primary caregiver for her severely autistic adult son, Daniel. While Jean finds great purpose in caring for Daniel, it tugs at her heart when she remembers him as he used to be. As a child, she recalls, "He was fine…. He did long division. He wrote in cursive. He was conversational." And now, she explains, "We have to help him wash. We have to help him shave. We have to help him wipe for a bowel movement. He can't communicate and he will never live any kind of normal life." Jean said that when her friend watched some videos of Daniel when he was much younger, "it affected her deeply emotionally." She told Jean, "I never knew how normal he was." Jean concludes, "Daniel needs help and I'm so thankful to be able to give that help to him."

The extraordinary love shown by caregivers like Mark and Jean is a special kind of love. It's deeper than parental love or romantic love, and even better than either of those. It's the love that the Bible calls *hesed* (*HEH-sed*). There is no English word that captures the full meaning of this Hebrew word. *Hesed* is a beautiful blend of love and loyalty, a faithful love that can be counted on. It is a deeply committed love that intervenes on behalf of the one who is loved.

We tend to think of love as a warm, fuzzy feeling. *Hesed* is not a feeling; it's choice-driven love that acts in the best interests of another person. It is love in action. It's what enables a caregiver to choose again and again to serve the person in their care.

It's important to point out that a heart full of *hesed* doesn't change the fact that caregiving is hard work. It doesn't take away the stress and weariness and challenges of caregiving. What *hesed* does do is answer the *why* question that sometimes comes into a caregiver's mind when the journey is hard: *Why am I doing this?* Because of love, that's why! Loyal, willing-to-go-above-and-beyond *hesed* explains why so many families choose to care for their loved one at home for as long as possible, even when it is difficult.

In our book for dementia caregivers, *Keeping Love Alive as Memories Fade,* my coauthors and I wrote this about *hesed:*

> We have used this word to describe the "gold standard" of dementia care—the loyal, merciful, intentional love that intervenes on behalf of loved ones and comes to their rescue. In antiquity, this

Hebrew word was used to describe the love of God Himself for humanity. There has never been a higher love than the *hesed* of God, and it is His love, many care partners tell us, that empowers them to love the person in their care so well.[5]

Since, as Jean said, "attitude is everything," you may want to think of your caregiving as a "trip to France" that God has asked you to take. Consider it a special, temporary assignment. And while you are on that trip, part of your assignment is, with God's help, to infuse your caregiving with *hesed,* the best possible kind of love.

The Downside of Caregiving

I'm going to take a guess—you didn't expect caregiving to be part of God's plan for your life, did you? Like Jean, Mark, and so many other caregivers, you may have had a very different plan in mind for this phase of your life. Maybe you were hoping for a job promotion that requires travel. Then you realized that travel would conflict with your caregiving responsibilities. Maybe you were thinking about furthering your education or moving to a different city or pursuing a hobby or a lifelong dream. But if those plans don't mesh well with caregiving, you may be struggling with mixed emotions, trying to decide if you should delay or abandon your goal so you can devote more time and energy to caregiving. And if you feel you have no choice about caregiving, you may be more than a little reluctant to embark on this unexpected detour.

Grief

If your scenario is anything like one of those, regardless of the love and loyalty that has brought you to this moment, you may be quietly grieving the loss of your plans. And you know what? It's okay to grieve. Grief is a normal response to loss or disappointment. Many aspects of caregiving can trigger grief for both you and for the person you now care for or will soon care for. Grief can be due to things in the present, or in the past, or even in the future.

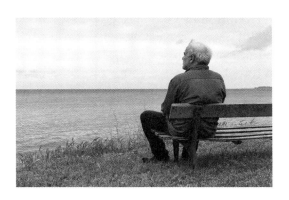

Grieving the Present

As a caregiver, you may have moments of grieving the present, because of small losses that happen due to your caregiving responsibilities ("Oh, I'm going to miss the birthday party!"). You may also grieve bigger things, such as:

- Seeing your loved one sick, impaired, or in pain.

- Recognizing more and more ways that caregiving has changed your life.

- Missing out on fun times with your friends or things you and your loved one used to do together but can no longer do. If you are caring for your spouse, you both might, for example, grieve missing the once-in-a-lifetime anniversary trip you had so looked forward to.

The person in your care may grieve multiple losses due to whatever created their need for your care. For example, their losses might include forced early retirement, no longer being able to drive, the need to sell their house, or finding a new home for a pet they love dearly but can no longer care for.

Grieving the Past

Sometimes present grief triggers unresolved grief from the past. Mark is experiencing this now as he cares for his wife, Michelle. As Michelle's condition worsens, she has more and more difficulty connecting emotionally with Mark. He grieves the slow loss of their once close relationship. This present grief has rekindled the grief he felt years ago when his first wife left their marriage. Right now, he says, "I'm having grief upon grief—grief from ten years ago along with a new grief."

Grieving the Future

Grieving a future loss is called anticipatory grief. Caregivers who expect their loved one's condition to get worse may grieve their decline before it occurs. Some may also grieve their loved one's death while that person is still living. If recovery is possible, a caregiver may live on a roller coaster of anticipatory grief: hopeful one day and sad the next.

THE STAGES OF GRIEF

Denial

Denial is the "this cannot be real" stage. A person in the denial stage can't yet wrap their head around what has happened. They may try to carry on just as if the loss had not really occurred. They may tell themselves and others, "I'm fine" or stay very busy so they won't think about the loss.

Anger

Anger is the "it's not fair" or "why did God let this happen?" stage. In this stage, a person might deal with their anger by blaming themselves or someone else. They may be argumentative, irritable, impatient, or sarcastic, sometimes toward people or things that aren't even connected to their loss, such as "the economy" or a slow cashier at the grocery store.

Bargaining

Bargaining is the "if," "if only," or "I should have" stage. A person in this stage is regretful, wishing to undo or repair what happened. They may make promises to themselves or God such as, "If my wife survives this surgery, I'll never argue with her about money again." They may brood over what might have changed the outcome: "If only I hadn't run out of gas, I would have been there when Mom fell. I should have stopped for gas when I had the chance."

Depression

It's normal to feel sad or "down" after a loss. In the depression stage, people may have trouble sleeping, feel unmotivated or hopeless, or cry. Crying is a normal response to sorrow. Shedding tears not only helps provide emotional relief but helps physically too. Crying lowers blood pressure and pulse rate and helps get rid of cortisol, the stress hormone.

The depression stage of grief is not the same as clinical depression, which is a medical condition. However, when the sadness of grief lingers on and on for a long time, it may deplete the brain's "happy chemicals" and result in clinical depression. When feeling "down" lasts more than a few weeks, it's best to see a doctor who may prescribe an antidepressant medicine. Many people find "talk therapy" helpful too—talking with a professional counselor about what's making you sad.

Acceptance

A person in the denial, anger, bargaining, or depression stage is still fighting against reality. Arriving at the acceptance stage doesn't mean they now like their circumstances. It means they have made peace with their "new normal." From a mindset of acceptance, they can now say along with the apostle Paul, "I have learned to be content whatever the circumstances" (Philippians 4:11). Acceptance allows them to face the future with courage and a positive attitude.

Jean said, "It's much easier to walk with the wind than against it." She explained, "With a disabled or mentally ill person, you have to come to a point where you say, 'You know, this is who they are, and God loves them exactly as they are.' I've come to see my son as a human being that is exactly as he is supposed to be right now." For Jean, acceptance "has been the most freeing thing."

No matter whether you are grieving the past, the present, or the future, there are three things everyone needs to remember:

- It's normal to grieve, not just when you experience loss, but also when reality doesn't turn out the way you wanted or expected.

- There is no wrong way to grieve. Each person works through grief in their own way and in their own time.

- Grief unfolds in stages. A grieving person may not cycle through the stages of grief in the tidy order listed above. It's also normal to cycle back through any stage before finally arriving at acceptance.

Caregiver Burden

As a family caregiver, it's important to realize that your sense of purpose and your love for the person in your care always exist alongside something known as *caregiver burden*.

Caregiver burden is the total weight of all the physical, mental, and emotional strain of caregiving. Caregiver burden can range from very slight to very severe, depending on the situation. The intensity of caregiving is measured by the number of hours of care provided and the number of tasks done during those hours.

The Caregiving in the US report found that:[6]

- Four out of 10 caregivers are in high-intensity situations. About the same number are in low-intensity situations, and the rest are in medium-intensity circumstances.

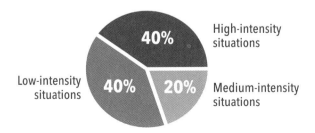

For employed caregivers …

- More than half report that they sometimes have to go in late, leave early, or take time off work in order to care for their loved one.

- About 14% have had to take a leave of absence.

- Some have stopped working altogether even though they still need the paychecks.

Family caregivers often do a lot more than meets the eye! The list of possible duties is long and varies widely with the situation. In addition to physically assisting the cared-for person, caregivers may do many other tasks, such as:

- Manage and give medicines.

- Make medical appointments and take the patient to them.

- Shop for groceries and make meals.

- Do household chores.

- Take care of bills and insurance paperwork.

- Contribute financially.

- Provide emotional and/or spiritual support.

Whatever is on a caregiver's to-do list is, of course, in addition to meeting their own personal, financial, and employment needs—and in some cases, the needs of a separate household and its members, which may include a spouse and/or young children. Think of caregiver burden as the total impact of caregiving on your life—your body, mind, emotions, faith, finances, job, and relationships. *As a family caregiver, you must continually stay aware of your level of caregiver burden.*

In the early stages of a chronic disease, or during a brief period of recovery after surgery, most family caregivers are able to manage just fine because the caregiver burden is light. When a cared-for person is physically or cognitively declining, many family caregivers bravely continue to shoulder the increasingly difficult load. They often do this sacrificially, out of a *hesed* kind of love and family loyalty, and often also because they cannot afford to pay for help.

Obviously, the sicker or more impaired a person becomes, the more care they will need. During the later stages of Alzheimer's or Parkinson's disease, for example, sometimes a caregiver's sacrificial love and family loyalty just aren't enough to bear up under the heavier caregiver burden. *This is why it's important to see every increase in caregiver burden as a waving yellow caution flag, reminding you to refocus on your self-care.* Failure to pay attention to increasing caregiver burden puts your wellbeing at risk, which may ultimately also risk the wellbeing of the person in your care.

Measuring Caregiver Burden

Experts say it is important to be extremely honest with yourself about the impact of caregiving on your life. You can measure your caregiver burden from time to time with a self-test called the Zarit Caregiver Burden Interview, also known as the Zarit Scale of Caregiver Burden. This screening tool is available in three versions:

- The full version, with twenty-two questions, provides the most specific assessment of burden. It has four scoring categories: little to mild burden; mild to moderate burden; moderate to severe burden; and severe burden.

- The twelve-item version rates burden as mild, moderate, or high.

- The simple version, with just four questions, produces scores between zero and sixteen.

You can find all three versions of the Zarit Caregiver Burden Interview on several websites (see the caregiver resources at the end of this book).

If you like, take a few minutes right now to complete the simple four-question Zarit assessment on the following page. Read the questions and circle the number that corresponds to how often you feel that way. To get your score, add the four numbers you chose. (In this assessment, *relative* refers to the person you are caring for.) If your score is eight or more, your caregiver burden is high. It's vital that you begin now to pay more attention to your self-care. The chapters ahead will give you suggestions about how to do that.

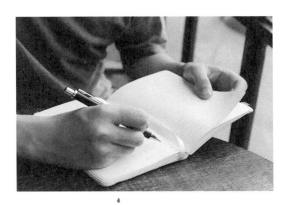

ZARIT SCALE OF CAREGIVER BURDEN

Do you feel that because of the time you spend with your relative, you don't have enough time for yourself?

Never	Rarely	Sometimes	Quite Frequently	Nearly Always
0	1	2	3	4

Do you feel stressed between caring for your relative and trying to meet other responsibilities for your family or work?

Never	Rarely	Sometimes	Quite Frequently	Nearly Always
0	1	2	3	4

Do you feel strained when you are around your relative?

Never	Rarely	Sometimes	Quite Frequently	Nearly Always
0	1	2	3	4

Do you feel uncertain about what to do about your relative?

Never	Rarely	Sometimes	Quite Frequently	Nearly Always
0	1	2	3	4

TOTAL SCORE: _____

The Importance of Self-Care

The unfortunate reality is that it's not always easy for busy caregivers to focus on their own mental and physical self-care. One in four caregivers say they find self-care difficult. This is most often true for those in high-intensity caregiving situations that require many hours of care. Others who find it difficult are those who live with the person they care for, have been providing care for more than a year, or had no choice about caregiving.[7]

Research also reveals that out of 100 caregivers:[8]

- 23 have skipped routine dental care more than once.

- 55 have skipped their own doctor appointments.

- 63 admit to poor eating habits.

- 21 rate their health as poor or fair; only half as many rate their health as excellent.

- Nearly 60 say their exercise habits got worse after becoming a caregiver.

- 25 to 50 are depressed.

Perhaps the most sobering finding to ever emerge from caregiver research was from the Caregiver

Health Effects Study which reported that elderly spouse caregivers who were strained by caregiving were 63% more likely to die within the next four years, compared to non-caregivers.[9] The study defined strained, at-risk spouse caregivers as those who were depressed, anxious, and "much less likely to get enough rest in general, have time to rest when they are sick, or have time to exercise." This study specifically focused on older caregivers (ages 66–96) who lived with the spouse they were caring for. Many were already dealing with an illness of their own.

Though you may be younger, healthier, and not living under the same roof as the person in your care, allow these findings to remind you that:

- Self-care is very important, regardless of your age or the intensity of your caregiving situation.

- Self-care is more difficult while caring for another person, so you must make it a high, non-negotiable priority.

- Self-care isn't selfish!

If you were to have the pleasure of talking with Mark about his caregiving experience, you would soon notice that he uses one word over and over. That word is *intentional*. According to the Merriam-Webster dictionary, *intentional* means "the determination to act in a certain way." It is also defined as "what one intends to do or bring about."

What I have learned from Mark is the importance of being intentional—"determined to act in a certain way"—in every aspect of caregiving. Mark is intentional about making an effort to connect emotionally with Michelle even when caregiving makes their lives busy and stressful. When he's tired at the end of the day, but there's still more to do, I wondered, how does he keep going? Not surprisingly, he said, "I turn on the intention button and get going. Till my head hits the pillow." When our conversation turned to self-care, I asked, "How do you take care of yourself while you're taking care of Michelle? Exercise, time with friends? Haircuts, dental and doctor appointments?" He said simply, "You have to be intentional" about finding time for yourself.

Mark is intentional about self-care because he understands why it's so necessary. It keeps his emotional, spiritual, and physical reserves from running out. It equips him to be the patient, loving, and truly *caring* caregiver he wants to be—and is.

Mark's best tip for caregivers, not surprisingly, is be intentional about taking good care of yourself.

CAREGIVING BY THE NUMBERS[10]

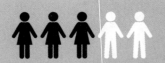

3 out of 5 caregivers
are women.

Caregivers by Age

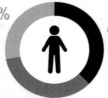

21%
age 65
or older

45%
age 44
or younger

34%
ages 45–64

Top 5 Reasons People Need a Caregiver

1. Aging
2. Difficulty getting around (mobility problems)
3. Alzheimer's disease or confusion
4. Recovery from surgery or wounds
5. Cancer

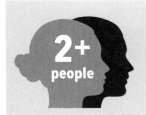

2+ people

About 1 in 4 caregivers provides care for 2 or more people.

4½ years

On average, caregivers provide a recipient with care for 4 ½ years.

3 out of 10 caregivers provide care for 5 years or more.

5+ years

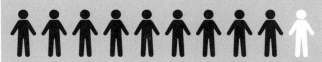

Nearly 9 out of 10 caregivers provide care for an adult relative.

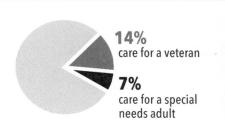

14%
care for a veteran

7%
care for a special needs adult

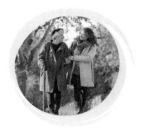

Chapter 2
Self-Care and the Stress of Caregiving

IT CAN'T BE SAID TOO OFTEN: CAREGIVING IS ONE OF the most important jobs you will ever do! As mentioned in the previous chapter, caring for a sick, injured, or aging loved one can bring wonderful new purpose and meaning to your life. It's work you can truly be proud of. That's the bright side of caregiving. At the same time, what's also true is that caregiving may be one of the most difficult jobs you'll ever have.

Caregiving can be very stressful work. Because many aspects of caregiver burden are related to stress, it's important to understand how stress affects your physical and emotional health.

Stress and Caregiver Burden

Many people are surprised to learn that both negative and positive experiences create stress.

- You might feel *eustress*, the good kind of stress, when you're playing a fun, competitive game with your friends or family.

- You would feel bad stress, known as *distress*, if it looks like you're about to be hit by a car.

The body responds to stress by mobilizing you to take action—fast. It equips you to either fight a threat or run away from it. That's why it's called the "fight or flight" response. In prehistoric times, danger was everywhere, and the fight or flight response was essential for survival. For example, if you were being stalked by a lion, the fight or flight response might have kept you off the dinner menu. But in the modern world, the fight or flight response is not always such a good thing.

Here's why:

Your body can't tell the difference between a minor stress and a life-threatening one. The stress of trying to win a competitive game hardly compares with the stress of being chased by a lion, but here's the thing—your body would respond the same way to both stresses. Unfortunately, the fight or flight response is an *overreaction* to many of the normal stresses of modern life. Missing your exit on the freeway, losing your cell phone, or a flooding basement can all cause the fight or flight response to kick in—and so can some of the challenges you face as a caregiver.

When something stressful happens, the body goes into emergency mode, quickly pumping out the stress hormones, adrenaline and cortisol. In response to adrenaline, the heart beats faster; blood pressure goes up; breathing speeds up, and the small airways in the lungs get wider. The muscles get tense. The pupils of the eyes even dilate to let in extra light. The other hormone, cortisol, sends extra glucose (sugar) into the blood stream to give you more energy. It also slows or alters the body systems that would not matter in a crisis, such as your immune, reproductive, and digestive systems. It's as if your whole body steps on a gas pedal to give you the burst of energy you need to deal with the crisis. Then, when the threat has passed, your body naturally "puts on the brakes," and in about twenty to thirty minutes, everything is back to normal.

Short periods of stress are not harmful. But when there is constant stress, your body can't go back to normal. With ongoing stress, cortisol keeps circulating in the blood to keep the fight or flight response turned on. This is when stress becomes harmful to health. Cortisol flows to every organ in the body, impacting health and well-being in many ways that show up as the physical and emotional symptoms of caregiver burden. Cortisol keeps on suppressing the immune system, making a person more likely to get sick. Anxiety, digestive problems, high blood pressure, poor sleep, weight gain, and headaches are just some of the health issues that can result when cortisol is continually released in response to ongoing stress. This is why high caregiver stress should *not* be ignored.

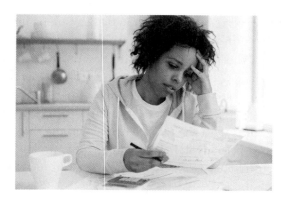

Recognizing Your Stress

As a cared-for person's health declines, caregiving can become more and more stressful as time goes on. Sometimes the need for more intense care arises suddenly, for example, if that person is injured in a fall. Other times, the need for more intense care increases very slowly as disease or dementia worsens over a long period of time. Caregiver burden that increases suddenly is easy to recognize—and it's often temporary. When it increases very slowly, you may not even notice that your load is getting a little heavier each day, until one day you realize it's become too heavy to carry. At that point, caregiver burden has opened the door to caregiver burnout. That's a road you do not want to go down! Burnout is a state of extreme exhaustion that can result when heavy caregiver burden has continued too long. To avoid burnout, you must take steps to manage your caregiver stress.

Before you can respond to increasing stress, however, you must first recognize it. To do that, you must pay close attention to the clues your body and emotions give you.

Listen to your body

- Is your blood pressure higher than it used to be?

- Are you getting more colds?

- Do you have muscle tension, headaches, or neck pain?

- Are you sleeping poorly?

- Are you gaining weight? Or losing weight without meaning to?

- Are you tired most of the time?

Listen to your emotions

- Do you feel "down" or depressed?

- Are you tense, nervous, or anxious?

- Are you overeating or drinking too much?

- Are you often irritable or angry?

- Do you feel the person you care for is unappreciative or asks too much of you?

- Do you feel alone or unsupported?

Some people are more sensitive to stress than others. That's why individuals may respond differently to the same stressful situation. It is thought that genes may play a role in each person's sensitivity to stress. Possibly, slight genetic differences make the fight or flight response overactive in some people and underactive in others. Past life experiences may also play a role. People who experienced abuse or neglect during childhood may have a stronger response to the stress of caregiving than others do. The same is often true of those who have been victims of a violent crime, survived an airplane crash, or served in the military or as first responders. Caregiver research reveals that women are more affected by the stress of caregiving than men. This is particularly true if a woman is taking caring of her husband, and especially if she cares for him in their own home. Women who care for a person with dementia or another condition that requires constant supervision or care also experience greater stress. According to the Alzheimer's Association, about 6 out of 10 dementia caregivers rate the emotional stress of caregiving as high or very high.[11]

If you have had traumatic life experiences, give yourself grace in the stressful moments of caregiving. Give yourself grace as well if you have other factors that can increase caregiver stress, such as:

- being socially isolated

- depression

- money problems

- caregiving for a high number of hours per week

- having no choice about being a caregiver

Responding Wisely to Your Stress

Now that you know about the fight or flight response and how stress and past life experiences factor into caregiver burden, put this knowledge to work for you! Pay attention to how you feel physically and emotionally. Don't ignore any clues that point to increasing stress. When your body or emotions alert you to rising stress, take action. Identify what you need most at that moment and then be intentional about seeking it. Any *yes* answer to the questions in the *Recognizing Your Stress* section above means it's time to begin seeking more support and care for yourself.

Sounds good, right? But there are two things that might stop you from taking care of yourself when you need it most:

1. **Exhaustion**
   If the intensity of your caregiving situation increases, the increase in mental and/or physical exhaustion may make it more difficult to devote time, energy, and money to your own self-care. Expect this challenge and don't let it rob you of the self-care you need.

2. **Guilt**
   It's not unusual for caregivers to feel guilty about taking care of themselves. The thinking

that drives guilt is often something like this: *The needs of the person I'm caring for are so much greater than mine! How can I possibly put my needs ahead of theirs?*

It can be hard to remember that taking care of yourself actually is, in the long run, also taking care of that other person. Do your best to believe that self-care isn't selfish. Rather, see it as an investment that will be repaid in a better quality of life for you and a better quality of care for your loved one. You deserve this and so does the person in your care. Give yourself permission to take good care of yourself!

My friend, Dr. Jo Cleveland, encounters caregivers on a regular basis in her work as a geriatric physician. She has realized that some caregivers need to hear someone *else* give them permission to take care of themselves. So she makes a point of telling them directly, "I'm giving you permission to take care of yourself while you take care of your mom." In response to those words, she says, "I've seen a lot of relief on faces." So, if it's difficult for you to give yourself permission to take care of yourself, you now have a doctor's permission to do so!

Another Way to Look at Self-Care

If you're still uncomfortable with making your own self-care a priority, maybe it will help to look at it a little differently. Consider these words of Jesus in light of caregiving:

> "Love your neighbor as yourself."
> MATTHEW 22:39

It's easy to relate the "love your neighbor" part of this verse to caregiving. But what about the "as yourself" part? We know, of course, that Jesus was not specifically talking about caregiving. But what if we consider this verse with caregiving in mind? What if the verse read like this: *Take care of your loved one in the same way you take care of yourself.* In other words, what if your self-care had to be the template for your loved one's care? How well-cared for would that person be?

Matthew Henry was an English theologian who lived from 1662 to 1714. In his beloved commentary on the Bible, he wrote this about the verse above:

> It is implied, that we do, and should, love ourselves. There is a self-love which is corrupt, and the root of the greatest sins, and it must be put off ... but there is a self-love which is

natural.... We must love ourselves, that is, we must have a due concern for the welfare of our own souls and bodies.[12]

Henry is saying that the kind of self-love that finds favor with God includes "a due concern for the welfare of our own souls and bodies." To say this another way, loving and caring for ourselves is a God-given stewardship. Merriam-Webster dictionary defines *stewardship* as "the careful and responsible management of something entrusted to one's care." This means that while you're on the caregiving journey, it's not only *okay* to take care of yourself— it's being a good steward of your life.

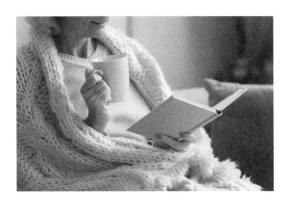

Coping with Your Stress

Every caregiver and every caregiving situation is unique. There is no "one size fits all" way to respond to the stresses of caregiving. Caregivers can, however, choose whether they will cope with their stress in healthy or unhealthy ways.

Unfortunately, not all caregivers deal with their stress in positive ways. One survey of over 1,000 long-term caregivers revealed that out of every 100 caregivers:[13]

- 32 coped by eating more.

- 22 shopped more.

- 27 worked more.

- 17 drank more alcoholic beverages.

The survey also revealed how caregivers coped in healthy ways. Out of 100 caregivers:

- 63 prayed or meditated.

- 51 spent time outdoors.

- 28 exercised more.

Managing caregiver stress can be challenging! However, much can be learned from caregivers who've found ways to deal with their stress in healthy, positive ways. Research on caregiving can be helpful too, highlighting what works for many people and what doesn't. The insights and tips below from Mark, Jean, and research can help you cope well with the common, stressful realities of caregiving.

1. Take Some Time for Yourself.

One of the most common stressful realities of caregiving is that it can be hard to find personal time. The demands of caregiving often mean that caregivers sacrifice time for themselves—and this is especially true if the caregiver lives under the same roof as the person in their care. This is the case for both Jean and Mark.

Jean said that her thirty-six-year-old autistic son "must always be in the direct sight" of a caregiver. "There's never a moment when he is out of sight, out of mind. Never." For this reason, Jean said, "I don't have a lot of private time. My life is structured, so I don't have a lot of flexibility." She is fortunate to have some evening caregivers or to tag team with Ryan at the end of the day. "At five o'clock or sometimes four o'clock," she said, "I'm done." With her physical and emotional reserves now running low, she typically retreats to an upstairs bedroom. Sometimes she tells her husband, "I'm going to have the door shut." She said, "I like my alone time."

Mark's situation is similar, except that there is no one else at home to take over his wife's care at the end of the day. When he compares caring for Michelle with caregiving in the past for his mother-in-law and his father, he notes an important difference. In both past situations, he said, "I could close the door and go home, leaving that person to be cared for by someone else." Now, he said, "I don't close the door and go home. I *am* home. I can never really, totally, close the door."

He explained, "I can't leave Michelle alone. That would be dangerous because of her risk for falls. She is unable to make her own meals or take her own meds because (due to Parkinson's) she drops them on the floor and can't pick them up." He said "I am on call 24/7. Consequently, phone calls are either not made or end quickly and tasks must wait to be completed. I don't have time to read very much or go outside."

Mark creates time for himself by arising around 5:30 a.m. to "make a cup of coffee and have a brief quiet time." In the evening, he is alone for about twenty-five minutes to take a shower. At night, he said, "When I close my eyes, I'm listening," always ready to respond. "If I hear my name, I'm right there for her." He said, "It's like sleeping with a baby in the room." He admits, "Having done this for nine months now, I'm in desperate need of a vacation."

Mark has some outside helpers who come for short periods of time during the week. During the few hours when Michelle has another caregiver, Mark visits his mother in her assisted living community or meets up with friends for lunch. Sometimes he works outside in the yard or goes to the gym where he is a member. He said, "You have to be intentional" about how to spend your free time. He said, "I could use more 'Mark time'."

Jean's Tip

- Make time at the end of the day when interruption is not permitted and enjoy whatever makes you feel happy.

Mark's Tip

- Pursue your favorite things to do, like gardening or reading, even if it's just for a short time and not every day.

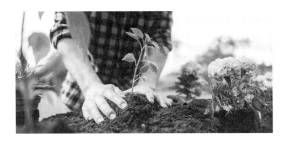

2. Realize that Friends or Family Members May Not Understand.

Research has found that friendships and family relationships can play an important role in caregiver well-being. Caregivers with strong friend networks feel less caregiver burden. Caregivers also feel less burden if their family members visit often. However, if friends and family members do not understand the challenges and the time crunch of caregiving, they may be unable to offer the kind of support the caregiver really needs.

Jean said, "I have a different kind of life and I love it when people reach out to me, even when I can't reach out to them. What I feel bad about is that I can't reach out to all my friends. I don't have time for a lot of small talk." This has sometimes resulted in an "I always call you; you never call me" situation that has caused hurt feelings. Jean explains, "That person wants me to take the time. They're feeling there's no reciprocity. But they don't understand my circumstances."

Fortunately, Jean also has friends who wonderfully "get it." She said, "Everybody in my life right now that is close to me, I have met because of my son. They understand that sometimes I just have to choose the higher priority at the moment." She added, "The thing that makes me cry are the people that don't 'get it'—

I don't love them any less. And what's interesting is that it's often your family."

Jean's Tips

- Share your life with those you know will understand. Not everyone does. Not everyone can.
- Let your friends know that you need to plan far in advance for fun times.

Mark's Tips

- Don't neglect your friendships. Treat yourself to phone calls and meals with your friends.
- Invite family members to come see the realities of caring for their loved one. Invite them to be a part of your caregiving plan.

3. Pay Attention to the Exhaustion Factor.

When I interviewed Mark for this book, part of our conversation went like this:

Me: What emotions has caregiving brought to the surface for you?

Mark: Exhaustion.

Me: Is that an emotion?

Mark: No, it's not. It's just a reality.

Me: Tell me about exhaustion.

He said, "It's mental and physical. When you miss your sleep, when you have to do more: give the bathroom help, give the meds—maintenance, the functional. I would rather sit down and just *be* ... and not function. Because the functional wears you out to the point where you're *spent*. At the end of the day, when I've had a really functional day, doing lots of functional things, the relational [connection with Michelle] is not there. You're both kind of depleted. But I still need to function with her until bedtime, until my head hits the pillow. You have to be intentional."

Despite the exhaustion, Mark said he doesn't feel burdened by caregiving. Rather, he said, "I feel *responsible*. The responsibility can be overwhelming."

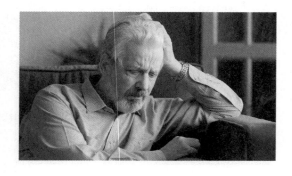

The C.A.R.E. Study found that 64% of caregivers say they feel tired. Of those that say they feel tired, 47% say they feel tired *often* and 17% say they feel tired *all the time*.[14]

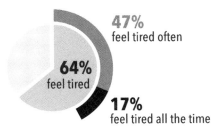

47% feel tired often

64% feel tired

17% feel tired all the time

Mark's Tips

- Begin with good rest: early bedtime and possibly a nap in the afternoon.
- Caregiving 24/7 is virtually impossible without assistance. Call on friends to come and sit for a few hours or hire a professional caregiver for a few hours a week.

4. Respond Wisely to Stressful Emotions.

Emotions are neither good nor bad. They're just powerful feelings that are often part of the grief process or coping with difficult circumstances. The C.A.R.E study leaves no doubt that caregiving can trigger your emotions.[15] The survey revealed the percentage of caregivers that reported feeling various emotions either often or all the time:

- **Sadness:** more than half (53%) often felt sad; 13% were sad all the time.

- **Anxiety:** nearly half (46%) often felt anxious; 12% were anxious all the time.

- **Guilt:** about a quarter of those surveyed (24%) often felt guilty; 6% felt guilt all the time.

- **Resentment:** about 16% felt resentful; 4% felt resentful all the time.

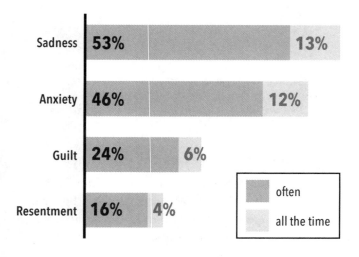

Resentment is concerning because if resentment is allowed to simmer for a long time, it can turn into anger.

Caregivers may feel resentful or angry if they:

- feel they have no choice about caregiving;

- lack help and support;

- feel unappreciated or taken for granted; or

- are exhausted, hungry, or sleep deprived.

Anger is one of the most powerful of all human emotions. It is a normal response to wrong treatment or injustice. It's not wrong to feel angry; it's just an emotion. But what we *do* with anger *can* be wrong. Anger can be destructive or even deadly if not handled wisely. That's why anger comes with a biblical warning: "In your anger, do not sin" (Ephesians 4:26). When caregiver burden is very high, and a caregiver is exhausted, overwhelmed, and lacks help from others, anger can erupt into verbal or physical abuse. It is vital for caregivers to resolve their angry feelings in a way that does no harm to the person in their care.

You can help guard against out-of-control anger by caring for yourself in three ways. When you feel your stress level rising, try the following quick and very simple way to suppress the fight or flight response.

1. Breathe in deeply for four seconds, making your belly expand as your lungs fill with air. Exhale slowly for eight seconds, so that breathing out takes twice as long as breathing in. Do this several times. When you breathe this way, the diaphragm moves, stimulating the calming function of the vagus nerve. This will slow your heart rate, lower your blood pressure, and help you feel more calm.

2. If slow, deep breathing isn't calming enough, choose a nondestructive way to discharge the energy of anger—punching a pillow, hammering nails, going for a run, or even cleaning your house. Any of these can help you deal with occasional anger or frustration. However, if you often feel anger or have simmering resentment, consider scheduling a visit with a mental health counselor soon. It's also vital for you to identify the kinds of help and support you need and take steps to find the help you need. (More about this in the next chapter).

3. Remember the word HALT, which stands for: **H**ungry, **A**ngry, **L**onely, **T**ired. Feelings of hunger, anger, loneliness, or tiredness are signals that your emotional and/or physical reserves are running low. When your reserves are low

you are more likely to *react* than *respond* in a stressful situation.

- When people *react,* their emotions are in control. What they say and do is driven by their emotions instead of by good judgment.

- When people *respond,* they are in control. They choose what they want to say or do.

It's always better to respond than to react! When your body signals you with feelings of hunger, anger, loneliness, or tiredness, pay attention. Before you react to a stressful circumstance, come to a HALT instead. Take slow, deep breaths, then respond with self-control to the stressful thing that is happening.

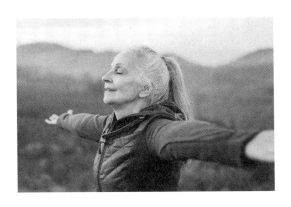

Jean's Tips

- Take time to feel your emotions; don't ignore them.

- Permit yourself to cry. It cleanses the soul. It is not wasted time.

- Be gentle with yourself when you make mistakes; we learn from them.

- Laugh at yourself. Give grace to yourself.

- Treat yourself the way you would treat a dear friend that you love.

- It takes practice, but live in the moment and don't allow worrisome thoughts to take you captive.

- Take a walk and think about what you see instead of what you need to do next.

5. Make Your Own Healthcare a Priority.

When you take the person you care for to one of their medical visits, it would be wonderful if the provider would turn to you, the caregiver, and say, "And how are *you* doing?" But studies show that this only happens about 13 times out of 100.[16] Most likely, you'll always be the "invisible patient" in the room. That's why you should be sure *your* healthcare providers know you are a caregiver. If they understand how caregiver stress can impact mental, physical, and emotional health, they might assess your caregiver burden. They may ask you the following questions.

- Do you feel that you're under a lot of stress?

- What do you do to relieve stress?

- Are you feeling "down" lately?

- Do your family and friends stay in touch with you?

If your healthcare providers have not talked with you about caregiver stress, consider completing one of the Zarit surveys and taking it with you to your next appointment. You can use your score to start a conversation about how you are feeling and what you need.

Make your annual physical exam and your regular dental checkups a high priority. One reason for checkups is to find and treat problems early. When a problem is found early, the chance of returning you to good health is highest. Regular checkups are doubly important if you have a chronic condition such as diabetes or high blood pressure. Even if you feel fine and have no medical issues, do not skip your checkups or preventive care, such as an annual flu shot. If you miss an appointment, always reschedule it. And ladies, I'm talking especially to you. Caregiver research reveals that women caregivers are less likely to get routine health screenings.

Do you need some extra motivation to keep up with your healthcare? Then just think about why your health matters to the person you take care of—in the unforgettable words of Dr. Seuss, "To the world you may be one person, but to one person you may be the world."

Jean's Tips

- Check your attitude daily by paying attention to what your body is telling you.
- Take deep breaths to relax the mind and release frustrations.
- Stretching exercises relax the muscles and can be done quickly and anytime.

Mark's Tips

- Look for a time to get some exercise: a brief walk outside or a short workout by video.
- Sit down to eat three meals a day and avoid nervous snacking.
- Take a daily multivitamin.

6. It's Okay If You Can't See the Finish Line.

Caregiving is often easier when everyone knows that care will only be needed for a short while. Caring for a skier while they wait for their broken leg to heal is far different than caring for someone with a chronic illness. When the broken leg is healed, the caregiver's life will likely go back to normal. But when a person has a chronic condition that only gets worse over time, caregiving is a long-term assignment with no finish line in sight. For many caregivers, this is discouraging. Mark said that seeing no end point is, for him, one of the hardest things about caregiving.

According to the Family Caregiver Alliance, on average, the typical caregiving arrangement lasts about four years. Dementia caregivers are the exception. They are more likely to provide care for five years or longer. In fact, some people with Alzheimer's disease live as long as twenty years after being diagnosed.[17]

In the C.A.R.E. Study:[18]

- Only about 2% of caregivers expected to provide care for less than 1 year.

- Most (71%) said they expected to be caregivers for up to 10 years.

- Another 18% anticipated providing care for 11 to 20 years.

- The remaining 8% thought they would be caregiving for even longer than 20 years.

2%	71%	18%	8%
Less than 1 year	1 to 10 years	11 to 20 years	More than 20 years

As long as medical research continues, there is always hope that many diseases will be cured in our lifetime. At present, however, it appears unlikely that Jean's son will be cured of autism or that Mark's wife will recover from Parkinson's disease. Thus, both Jean and Mark expect to continue caring for their loved one for as long as they and that person both live. How do they keep going when caregiving has no end in sight?

They both say it's all about perspective. For them, it is as Jean said earlier: "attitude is everything." Like so many "long haul" caregivers, they each feel that their role is a deeply meaningful expression of the *hesed* kind of love.

- Jean said, "I think the job of a caregiver is holy and my views are rooted in that belief. I do not see it as a burden but as a blessing. We are blessed to be given the life of helping the helpless."

- Mark said, "You don't know when your caregiving will stop, so you press on. Sometimes I don't know if I can take another step. Then a joy nugget comes along."

A joy nugget, Mark explained, is anything "that keeps us pressing on." It could be a happy memory, a song, the kindness of a friend, a verse of Scripture—whatever helps to "carry you through the unending, not-knowing-what's-next-events" of caregiving. Because his wife's disease is presently incurable, Mark said he and Michelle want to make the most of the time they have together. "It's going to get worse. We both know that. And so we create nuggets of joy in our relationship too, to not miss a moment." Together, Mark and Michelle have adopted this mindset: "Neither of us would have chosen this. But we've been given it. And we will not let it steal our joy."

Jean's Tips

- Remind yourself that God chose you for this time and this moment with this person.
- Find things to be thankful for each day.

THREE HAPPINESS BOOSTERS
FOR CAREGIVERS

1. Laugh Often.

Laughter reduces tension and anxiety, relaxes the muscles, increases energy, lowers bad cholesterol, and even helps strengthen the immune system. And here's the best part: your body can't tell the difference between genuine laughter and "fake" laughter. You get the benefits no matter why you're laughing. So laugh when things are funny, and even when they're not, go ahead and laugh anyway. It's really good for you.

2. Stay Flexible.

Whether the person in your care is recovering or declining, their needs will change over time. While it's helpful to have a set daily routine, a flexible approach to caregiving makes it easier to adapt as needs change.

3. Grow Your "Attitude of Gratitude."

According to behavioral research, gratitude is linked to greater satisfaction in life, optimism, empathy, and forgiveness. Experts also say that gratitude is a major key to resilience. Resilience is the ability to bounce back when difficulties knock you down. If the stresses of caregiving have you feeling less than grateful right now, you can grow your gratitude by keeping a gratitude journal. At least once a week, write in your journal about one thing you can choose to be grateful for. In time, these seeds of gratitude will sprout, helping you avoid the negativity and anxiety that threaten the happiness of many caregivers.

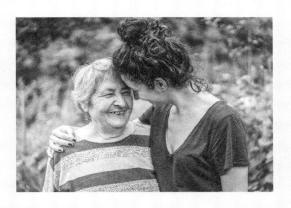

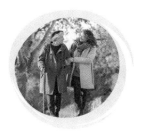

Chapter 3
Building Your Caregiving Team

FULL-TIME CAREGIVING IS NOT A JOB FOR JUST ONE person. Rather, it is, as my friend Dr. Ed Shaw says, "a team sport." If anyone understands the wisdom and necessity of taking a team approach to caregiving, it's Ed. His wife, Rebecca, was diagnosed with early onset Alzheimer's disease when she was just fifty-three years old. Ed, while still employed, was her primary caregiver for nine years. In the final two years of Rebecca's life, there were seventeen people on her and Ed's care team. That team consisted of their three daughters, other family members, some paid caregivers, good friends, and a pastor. In his book, *The Dementia Care-Partner's Workbook,* Ed recalls, "Everyone on the team came to our home and was involved in supporting her or me, physically, emotionally, and spiritually, on a daily, weekly, or monthly basis. Some were involved by their own choosing, others because I asked."[19]

Do you need a team like Ed's?

If you're thinking *oh yes!* then you're ready to start building your team. But if you're not sure, then there's a different question to answer first …

Are You a Care *Partner* or a Care *Giver*?

Though many people use the terms *care partner* and *caregiver* to mean the same thing, I think it's helpful to distinguish between them. If you are temporarily caring for someone recovering from surgery or an accident or caring for someone in the early stages of a chronic illness, your caregiver burden is likely low or very low. That's partly because, to some degree, the cared-for person can be involved in their own care. They can make decisions. They can do many things for themselves. They can, hopefully, also express appreciation to you for what you do for them. Whether they are slowly recovering or slowly declining from an illness, right now it's not exhausting or excessively time consuming to care for them. In situations where the care is shared to some degree, you and that person are *care partners*.

If you are caring for an elderly person or someone with a chronic illness, such as Parkinson's disease or Alzheimer's disease, at some point partnering will no longer be possible. As that person continues to decline and you must do more and more, care *partnering* gradually fully transitions to care *giving*. Sometimes, as with Jean and her autistic son, care partnering is not possible at any point. If your caregiver burden is moderate, heavy, or severe, you're truly a care *giver*.

If you are a care *partner*, and your caregiver burden is low, you may not need a team—at least not right now. If the person you care for is more likely to decline than to recover, use this time to think about the kind of team you'll soon need. If you are a care *giver*, and you know your caregiver burden is increasing, now is the time to start recruiting your team. It's important that you don't put this off too long because, as you now know, unrelenting stress puts you at risk for burnout. If you are willing to risk burnout there is something you need to know. Believe it or not, there's something worse than caregiver burnout.

Compassion Fatigue

People who work in high-stress jobs such as healthcare, law enforcement, or mental health counseling must constantly engage with those in emotional distress, pain, or traumatic circumstances. The constant exposure to highly stressful, compassion-triggering situations can result in something called compassion fatigue. Compassion fatigue weakens a person's empathy. It makes those in a position to help lose their sensitivity to others. Worse, they become indifferent to their suffering. This shutting down of compassion is a means of emotional self-preservation. This same desensitizing process can happen to caregivers who push themselves past their burnout point.

Compassion fatigue is a more serious concern for caregivers than for those in high stress occupations. Employers help their workers cope and regroup by providing them with counseling services, mental health days, paid time off for vacations or illness, and peer support. Caregivers have none of these resources—unless they put them in place themselves. And that's exactly why you need to create a team to surround and support you emotionally and in practical ways. You deserve a team to help you carry on the important, wonderful, difficult—and yes, sometimes heroic—job of caregiving!

Some (Very Bad) Reasons Why Caregivers Don't Create a Team

When caregiving is becoming too much for a caregiver to handle alone, it's wise and entirely reasonable to reach out for some help. Yet some caregivers won't. Even some who resent not having enough help resist seeking it. Those who continue to try to do it all, all by themselves, usually do so for one of these three reasons:

- They believe no one else can do what's needed as well as they can.

- They believe no one else *should* help because it's their sole responsibility.

- Pride. They are embarrassed or ashamed to admit they need help.

If any or all of these reasons are keeping you from recruiting the help you need, may I say as kindly as possible, none of these are good reasons for refusing to seek help. You've done many things through the years to help other people. Now it's your turn to be on the receiving end. Be wise and gracious and humble enough to seek and accept help from others. As my friend Ed wrote in his book for caregivers, "Most of us are much better at serving than at being served. Now is the time for you to receive the grace others extend to you."[20]

There is also a fourth reason why some caregivers don't reach out for help:

- They are secretly worried about being "replaced" by their helpers.

If that's your worry, consider this: if you allow others to assume some of your duties, you'll have more time to spend *with* your loved one instead of doing things *for* them. You'll be able to focus more on the relationship while others focus on the tasks. As my friend Dr. Jo Cleveland reminds caregivers, "No one else can be his wife, but someone else can get the groceries."

Don't try to go it alone. Caregiving really *is* a team sport. Let's start building your team!

> "Two are better than one, because they have a good return for their labor: If either of them falls down, one can help the other up."
>
> ECCLESIASTES 4:9-10

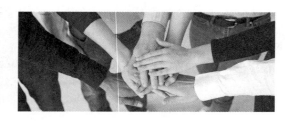

How to Build Your Team

You're the team captain, and as team captain, your first job is to determine exactly what kinds of help you need. Others may offer suggestions and opinions, but you are the only one who truly knows what's needed. Think about the kinds of practical help you need. Practical help is about tasks. It includes all the specific things on your caregiver to-do list that someone else could help you with. It also includes the other responsibilities that require your time and energy that others could assist with, such as caring for your home or children.

With a pen and four sheets of blank paper in hand, find a quiet, comfortable place where you can thoughtfully create some lists. Then follow these steps:

Step 1

On three of the sheets of paper, write one of these titles:

- Daily
- Weekly
- Monthly

List every caregiving and household task you now do and place each task on one of the papers. Seeing all you do written down in black and white will show

you how much is really on your plate. For example,
your lists might look something like this:

DAILY

- Wake John and help him dress
- Help John shave
- Make breakfast
- Clean up kitchen
- Give morning meds
- Make beds
- Assist John with stretching routine
- Make lunch
- Give mid-day meds
- Load wheelchair into car
  (Monday, Wednesday, Friday)
- Take John to physical therapy
  (Monday, Wednesday, Friday)
- Back at home, unload wheelchair
  (Monday, Wednesday, Friday)
- Help John into bed for nap
- Set John up at the computer or TV
- Make dinner

- Load dishwasher
- Help John shower
- Give evening meds
- Help John get ready for bed

WEEKLY

- Make grocery list
- Shop for groceries
- Change sheets
- Laundry
- Get gas
- Mow lawn
- Clean bathrooms

MONTHLY

- Take John to appointment with Dr. Browning
- Take John to appointment with Dr. Gray
- Fill prescriptions at pharmacy
- Pay bills
- Work on insurance forms

WEEKLY
- Make grocery list
- Shop for groceries
- Change sheets
- Laundry
- Get gas
- Mow lawn

Step 2

Circle or highlight the tasks that someone else could help you with. Put a check mark beside the tasks you would most like help with—the tasks you least enjoy doing or that burden you most. On the example lists above, could someone else...

- assist John with his stretching routine one or two days a week?

- shop for groceries?

- mow the yard?

- change the sheets and clean bathrooms?

- take John to his physical therapy session one or two days a week? Or to his monthly doctor visits?

- help John shower and get ready for bed a few evenings each week?

- spend a few hours with John one day a week to give you some personal time?

- pick up prescriptions?

WEEKLY
- Make grocery list
- Shop for groceries ✔
- Change sheets
- Laundry
- Get gas
- Mow lawn ✔

Step 3

After you've identified the tasks others could help with, it's time to brainstorm about who might be able to help. On your fourth sheet of paper, list all the possibilities: family members, friends, neighbors, members of your faith community, and if you can afford it, a house cleaning service, lawn service, and/or paid caregivers. Paid caregivers can often assist with tasks such as bathing and grooming, overnight care, or helping with laundry or light housekeeping.

Think about the personalities, skills, and availability of the people in your life. Match your potential helpers with the tasks.

- Might some friends of the person in your care be willing to spend a few hours with him or her once a week?

- Could your son mow the lawn?

- Could your next-door neighbor take the person to some appointments?

- Are there members of your faith community who might help with housework?

- Could a friend pick up prescriptions or run occasional errands?

WEEKLY

- Make grocery list
- Shop for groceries ✔ ← NEIGHBOR
- Change sheets
- Laundry
- Get gas
- Mow lawn ✔ ← SON

Step 4

Once you know what kind of practical help you need, and you have a list of potential helpers, you're ready to reach out. You can text, email, or write a letter, of course, but a phone call or a one-on-one conversation may be best. Speaking with the person gives them an opportunity to ask questions and chat with you a bit. No matter how you choose to reach out, simply share:

- The condition or illness of the person in your care.

- That you're their (full-time/part-time) caregiver.

- That you're putting together a team of people to help and support you.

- That you're wondering if they could help with _____.

Don't expect that everyone on your list will be able or willing to help. Be prepared to hear, "I'm sorry, I wish I could, but..." There are many good reasons why people may be unable to join your team. Enjoy each conversation, and when someone says *no,* don't think of it as a wasted call. Instead, remember that because you reached out, one more person is now aware of your situation. Even though the "no" people can't help in tangible ways, some of them might turn out to be great encouragers! Others might be willing to help, but maybe only once a month or from time to time. For everyone who can help on a regular basis, make a schedule and plug your daily, weekly, and monthly volunteers into it.

After you've contacted everyone on your list, if you still lack help, Jean would encourage you to "seek out resources in the community. There is a lot of help out there." She is thinking of things like the Meals on Wheels program, adult day care programs, respite care programs for parents of children with special needs, and local volunteer organizations. One such organization near the town where I live is the Shepherd's Center, an interfaith organization that serves older adults and their caregivers. Shepherd's Center volunteers provide transportation to medical appointments, shop for groceries, make friendly home visits, provide insurance and Medicare counseling, and even do minor home repairs. Like many organizations across the country, the Shepherd's Center also offers caregiver support groups and the Powerful Tools for Caregivers course. There are dozens of Shepherd's Centers in towns all across the United States. To find out if there is one near you, go to shepherdcenters.org and click on "Search the Network." (Also see the caregiver resources in the back of this book.)

Perseverance is the key to finding helpful community and government programs. Jean said, "I remember making phone call after phone call after phone call. One phone call led to another. Persist because all phone calls are useful. Ask questions: *Can you guide me? Do you know of anybody I could call?* There's never a call that isn't worth it. I'll never forget one call when I was seeking help for my son. The lady on the phone said 'There's a long list for autism money. I'm sorry, ma'am, you'll be way down on the list.' I said, 'That's so hard. Because I have a daughter with the same thing.' The woman said, 'Oh, you have *two*.' All of a sudden they got me on the list! I had no idea that having two was meaningful."

Jean's persistence paid off. She eventually did find the resources her family needed. Today, more than twenty years later, the necessary help is still in place. The family has helpers who come to their home several times a week and assist Daniel with routine needs, such as showering, and others who take Daniel on outings in the community. Jean is grateful to now be able to say, "I'm not the only one." Her advice to other caregivers is "Persist until you find the help you need."

Caregiver Tip

- Express gratitude to those who help you. Say thank you. Make requests, certainly, but don't make demands. If someone on your team feels you are unappreciative or demanding, they may stop helping. Don't take for granted anyone who steps up to help, including your own family members.

Finding Social and Emotional Support

We all need other people. But sometimes we don't reach out to others unless we are compelled to do so by circumstances we can't handle alone. If that sounds like you, and you're now willing to reach out to others because of your caregiving needs—good for you! *Good* because experts say that caregivers with strong social and emotional support systems are better able to weather the stresses of caregiving.

Caregiving can be a very lonely experience. Yet, how much "people time" we each need varies from person to person. It all depends on what naturally energizes and invigorates you. If you're more of a natural introvert, you may crave more personal "down time," time alone to think, rest, read, or pray. If you're more of a natural extrovert, you may crave more time in the company of others.

But what if neither *introvert* nor *extrovert* really describes you? What many people don't know is that there is a third category! If you sometimes recharge by being alone and other times recharge by being with people, you're probably an *ambivert*. An ambivert has both extroverted and introverted characteristics. Ambiverts have a flexible personality that can be either reserved or outgoing, depending on the situation. If you're an ambivert, you have a lot of company. It is estimated that nearly two-thirds of the population may be ambiverts.

All caregivers need both time alone and time with others. You know yourself best. Which energizes you most: solitude, social interaction, or sometimes one and sometimes the other? Seek the balance of time alone and time with others that best meets your needs and is possible in your circumstances.

Caregivers often have very little time for themselves. When "me time" is hard to come by it's important to use it wisely. Give thought to:

- What truly nurtures you?

- What best relaxes you?

- What small pleasures can you enjoy in a brief snippet of time? Some ideas:

  - Watch the sky at sunrise or sunset

  - Stretch parts of your body

  - Ponder one verse of Scripture

  - Savor the aroma of fresh coffee or flowers

Social and emotional support is found in nurturing relationships. But not all relationships are nurturing! That's why *who* you spend your limited time with matters. The words and attitudes of others can either encourage and energize you or discourage and drain you. To thrive as a caregiver, you need patient, empathetic, nonjudgmental support and understanding from people you trust and can talk openly with. Think about your relationships and consider each person's impact on your happiness and well-being:

- Who makes you laugh?

- Whose company do you enjoy?

- Who encourages you?

- Who makes you feel capable? Loved? Relaxed?

- Who listens to you without judgment or criticism?

- Who can you speak freely with?

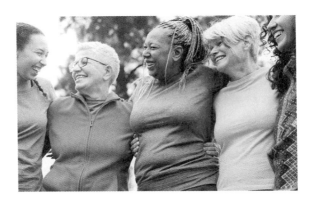

Many caregivers find it very helpful to be part of a caregiver support group. Since everyone in the group is there for the same reason, participants often enjoy a kind of camaraderie that is hard to find with people who are not caregivers themselves. However, people's social and support needs differ. Not every caregiver wants or needs to be in a support group, and not everyone has the time and energy to participate in one. People may also need different types of support at different times in their caregiving journey. Here are two different points of view from caregiver moms with autistic sons.

In an article for *Psychology Today*, writer Kimberly Grosso shares:

> One of the best pieces of advice given to me from my son's diagnosing physician was to join a local autism support group. It wasn't until I actually joined the group did I really start to appreciate what an invaluable resource it was. Talking with other parents who also have children on the spectrum helps parents to cope and express the stress they are experiencing. Because local support groups allow parents to make contact with other parents in the area, they are often one of the best places to get recommendations about local services and schools.[21]

Jean, who has shared much of her caregiving journey in this book, feels differently:

> As far as being in a support group, my answer would be *no*. And I'll tell you why. In my free time, I have to totally get away from caregiving. *Totally*. I have to have my mind on watching the woodpeckers and hearing the birds and taking my walks. Breathing the air and touching my toes so I can stay in shape and have that part of a normal life. Caregiving is a big part of my life, but it's also just a part. I don't want it to *be* my life.

Would a caregiver support group be helpful to you? Here are two more points to consider:

Since the COVID-19 pandemic, being with other people "virtually" online has become a normal part of life. However, research has brought to light the fact that caregivers who participate in online support groups still feel very alone. While being with others virtually is definitely better than having no contact at all with other caregivers, people seem to have a need to be in the physical presence of others. If you have a choice, opt for in-person support.

If you don't feel the need for a support group, but you do have the time and energy to participate in one, you may want to consider starting a group or helping to lead one. If you are a seasoned caregiver, your experience, insights, and presence might make a difference for someone new to caregiving or struggling to bring their life into balance.

Enlisting Your Team for Mini-breaks

It's not always easy to arrange for a whole day away from caregiving. But it may not be nearly as hard to arrange for an occasional mini-break, just some brief time off in the middle of the day to do "your thing," whatever that may be on a given day.

Do you have trustworthy friends and family members who've said to you, "If there's ever anything I can do, just let me know"? If those people are not already on your team and helping in some other way, keep a list of their names and phone numbers handy. When you're feeling exhausted or overwhelmed and can't seem to find even a few minutes for yourself, reach for that list. This is the time to call!

Reaching out spur-of-the-moment, you'll probably find whoever you call having their own busy day and unable to help. But if you're lucky enough to connect with a friend who just happens to be available right then, ask them to come over and take your place for just an hour. That's enough time for you to take a short nap, or go for a walk or a run, or simply sit on a park bench and breathe some fresh air.

Mini-breaks won't be possible in every situation. Sometimes a willing person just lives too far away to make a very short visit practical. Sometimes no one you know has a schedule that's flexible enough to come give you a break. When no one can step up, could you hire a professional caregiver for a few hours a week to give yourself a break?

If mini-breaks are possible, and you find them helpful, plan ahead with friends or family to line up some for the weeks ahead. If you're best recharged in the company of others, you may be able to use a two-hour mini-break to connect with someone socially. Ideas: take a walk with a neighbor, attend an online or in-person support group, or meet your sibling for coffee.

Caregiver Tip

- If you've asked a friend or family member for two hours of their time, honor that time commitment. Don't drive or walk so far that you can't be back when you said you would.

Counseling Is Sometimes Helpful.

Caregiving doesn't always mesh well with family dynamics. If your caregiving situation is complicated because of difficult family issues, counseling may be helpful. A professional counselor may be able to provide some of the insights and guidance you need in situations such as these:

You are taking care of a parent or family member you do not have a happy history with.

In an ideal world, every family would be loving, and every child would grow up in the security and nurture of *hesed.* But in this fallen and complex world, that's not always the case. If you are responsible for the care of a family member who has failed you or harmed you in the past, you may have painful memories that now interfere with your ability to care for them. Perhaps you're not sure what it would take—or whether you are even willing—to repair your relationship with the person in need of a caregiver. A counselor may be able to help you sort through these difficult issues.

None of your siblings or extended family supports or helps you.

If you are caring for a family member, it's only reasonable to expect siblings or others closely related to that person to carry part of the load. When they don't, it may be hard to handle the disappointment or resentment you may feel. You may also wonder how you should respond to what one caregiver described as her family's "excusing themselves from the journey." If you receive little or no encouragement or practical help from your family, it's definitely time to build your caregiving team—and to consider adding a counselor to it.

You're caring for someone who doesn't appreciate what you do for them.

One daughter who is her parents' caregiver said, "I am experiencing anger. And I know it stems from hurt.... My parents are ungrateful. There is *no* appreciation for what I do." If you, too, feel trapped by the obligation to provide care for someone who is unkind or unappreciative of the sacrifices you make in order to take care of them, perhaps a counselor could offer helpful guidance and perspective.

Conversations with a trained, licensed professional counselor are confidential, so a counseling office is a safe place to talk openly about your family issues. If your employer has an Employee Assistance Program (EAP), short-term counseling may be available to you for free. If not, some counseling practices have a sliding fee scale that is based on income.

Knowledge Boosts Confidence.

You've probably heard the saying, "knowledge is power." This is true when it comes to caregiving. The more you know about the condition of the person you care for, and about the natural progression of their disease, the fewer surprises you'll have. Understanding their condition, knowing what's normal and what's not, and what to expect, will make you a more confident caregiver. Educating yourself about the condition or disease of the person in your care is one way to make caregiving just a little bit easier. Here's how:

- **Read.**
  Ask the person's healthcare team for brochures, booklets, recommended websites, or videos that will help you learn more.

- **Ask.**
  Make a list of your questions and bring it with you when you take the person to their next medical appointment. Ask the doctor or a nurse what you'd like to know. If you're in a caregiver support group, talk with any others who provide the same kind of care as you do.

God Is Your Ever-Present Help.

The stress and busyness of caregiving can really weigh you down spiritually. But that doesn't have to happen. Psalm 46:1 says, "God is our refuge and strength, an ever-present help in trouble." You can take this verse personally. God wants to be your refuge, give you strength, and be there for you as an ever-present help in all the caregiving challenges you face.

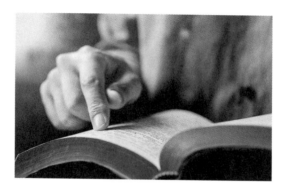

If you are a Christ-follower, invite him into your daily caregiving adventures. If you're not sure what all this is about, but you'd like to know more, go to cru.org and click on "How to know God." To grow a deeper connection to God, as Mark would say, you have to be *intentional* about it. If you've never read the Bible, start with the book of John in the New Testament.

If you don't have a Bible, you can read it online at the Bible Gateway website (biblegateway.com). If you already do read the Bible, you may find it meaningful to also read a daily devotional book, especially one written for caregivers. In the caregiver resources at the end of this book, you'll find a list of websites, books, and organizations to help you deepen your connection to God.

You can find strength in knowing that the Lord has not left you alone on your caregiver journey! He truly wants to be your "refuge and strength, an ever-present help."

"Trust in the LORD with all your heart and do not lean on your own understanding. In all your ways acknowledge Him, and He will make your paths straight."

PROVERBS 3:5–6 NASB

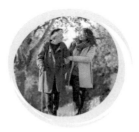

Afterword
When Caregiving Must Change

IF THE DAY SHOULD ARRIVE WHEN YOUR LOVED ONE'S needs exceed your ability to meet them, then what?

For many families, the hardest decision they ever have to make is when or if to place their loved one in a group home, memory care unit, or skilled nursing facility. But sometimes no decision has to be made— because circumstances make the decision for you. This is how it happened for Jean and her family.

As you know, Jean had been the primary caregiver for both of her autistic children since her daughter was twelve years old and her son was fifteen. She continued caring for them as adults, both still at home until one eventful day just a few years ago.

"One day my daughter was just not talking right," Jean recalls. "I couldn't follow her conversation. And then she started to get edgy. I saw that she was in psychosis." (A person in psychosis has lost touch with reality and may hallucinate and have difficulty speaking coherently.) "I called the doctor and I said, 'I'm not sure what to do.'" When the doctor, a psychiatrist, started telling Jean what to do, she responded, "You don't understand. If my total focus is on my daughter, how am I going to be able to take care of my son?" At that point they called an ambulance.

Jean's oldest daughter, a medical doctor, then got involved. She said, "Mom, this is too much for you." And Jean agreed.

Looking back on that eventful day, Jean now says,

> I could take care of *one* of them. But when one of them was decompensating—having this disconnected thinking—I couldn't take care of them both. My older daughter took over at that point. She found a supervised care residence for her sister. And that's how my younger daughter ended up not living with us anymore. I just could

never ever have made that decision—to tell my daughter, "You're going to have to live somewhere else." I just couldn't. So it took a crisis. That's the beautiful thing about it. Someone might say, 'How could that be beautiful?' But look how God intervened. Something happened that could have been really bad and now my daughter is in a good place where she needs to be. She's in a house with a roommate and she has 24/7 supervision. And she's happy. Sometimes it's a crisis that moves us in the direction that God has for us.

When there is no crisis that forces a quick decision, families have time to ponder and discuss the options. What would be best for the person who now needs more intense care? What would be best for the family, considering the cost of care and how far away from family the person would be? Even when everyone agrees on why and where to relocate their family member, it can still be a very emotional and difficult decision to make. One reason this is often a hard decision is because it can trigger feelings of guilt.

Dr. Jo Cleveland has counseled many caregivers who are wrestling with these guilt feelings:

> I have often heard caregivers say, "But I promised I would never put him in a nursing home!"

I respond by saying something like this: "I'm sure that when you said those words what you probably meant was that you would take care of him in your home for as long as it was safe and possible. It's no longer safe. And so it's no longer possible. Now you need to find what the next safe situation is."

If you are facing this difficult decision now, or if you face it later in your caregiving journey, let Dr. Cleveland's words give you confidence as you choose the "next safe situation" for the person in your care. If feelings of guilt arise, acknowledge them, but push past them to do what's best for your loved one. Keeping him or her safe and ensuring their best care is the most loving thing you can do for them, now and always.

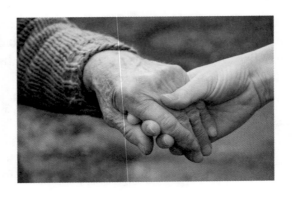

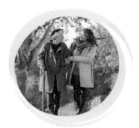

Resources for Caregivers

Caregiver Self-Care

Zarit Burden Interview, full twenty-two-item version
www.agingcare.com/documents/Caregiver_Burden_
Assessment.pdf

National Respite Network https://archrespite.org

Powerful Tools for Caregivers Classes (by state)
www.powerfultoolsforcaregivers.org

Caregiving Information and Support

Caregiver Action Network www.caregiveraction.org

Family Caregiver Alliance www.caregiver.org

Caregiving Research

Caregiving in the US 2020, AARP Research Report
download PDF from www.aarp.org/ppi/info-2020/
caregiving-in-the-united-states.html

For Cancer Caregivers

National Cancer Institute Resources for Caregivers
www.cancer.gov/resources-for/caregivers

For Caregivers of Older Adults

AgingCare.com www.agingcare.com

Area Agencies on Aging (listed by state)
www.agingcare.com/local/area-agency-on-aging

Shepherd's Centers of America
www.shepherdcenters.org

For Spouse Caregivers

Well Spouse Association wellspouse.org

For Dementia Caregivers

Alzheimer's Association
www.alz.org/help-support/caregiving

*The Dementia Care-Partner's Workbook: A Guide for
Understanding, Education, and Hope* by Edward
G. Shaw, MD, MA (Companion Press, 2019)

Grace for the Unexpected Journey: A 60-Day Devotional for Alzheimer's and Other Dementia Caregivers by Deborah Barr (Moody Publishers, 2018)

Keeping Love Alive as Memories Fade: The 5 Love Languages and the Alzheimer's Journey by Deborah Barr, Edward G. Shaw, and Gary Chapman (Northfield Publishing, 2016)

Resources for Spiritual Growth

YouVersion Bible App for your tablet or phone
www.youversion.com/the-bible-app

CRU www.cru.org

Bible Gateway (read the Bible for free online)
www.biblegateway.com

Charles Stanley's 30 Life Principles
www.intouch.org/topics/30-life-principles

Beyond Suffering Bible by Joni Eareckson Tada (Tyndale, 2016)

Acknowledgments

Some very special people played a big part in creating this little book. My sincere thanks goes first of all to my two-member "panel of experts," Jean and Mark, the full-time caregivers who graciously shared their caregiving stories with me. Jean and Mark are not their real names, and a few identifying details were changed to protect their families' privacy. Jean and Mark, thank you both so much for all you shared to encourage and help other caregivers. I want to thank you, and Jean's older daughter as well, for reading the manuscript and offering great feedback and suggestions.

I want to also thank Jo Cleveland, MD, and Claire Shaw for reading the manuscript. Jo, thank you for sharing your professional expertise and allowing me to pass some of your comments along to readers. Claire, thank you for sharing from your own personal experience as a dementia caregiver.

Book writing, like caregiving, is also best as a "team sport," and I'm glad all of you were on my team!

Notes

1   *Caregiving in the United States 2020, Executive Summary.* Washington, DC: AARP and National Alliance for Caregiving; 2020.

2   *Long term care in America: Expectations and realities.* Chicago: The Associated Press and National Opinion Research Center; 2014.

3   *Caregiving in the United States 2020.* Washington, DC: AARP and National Alliance for Caregiving; 2020.

4   *2019 C.A.R.E. Study.* Milwaukee: Northwestern Mutual; 2019.

5   Deborah Barr, Edward G. Shaw, and Gary Chapman, *Keeping Love Alive as Memories Fade: The 5 Love Languages and the Alzheimer's Journey* (Northfield Publishing, 2016), 204.

6   *Caregiving in the United States 2020* and *Executive Summary.*

7   *Caregiving in the United States 2020.*

8   Caregiver Statistics Caregiver Action Network, https://www.caregiveraction.org/resources/caregiver-statistics.

9   Richard Schulz and Scott R. Beach, "Caregiving as a Risk Factor for Mortality. The Caregiver Health Effects Study," *Journal of the American Medical Association* 282 (23) (December 15, 1999): 2215–2219.

10   These numbers are from *Caregiving in the United States 2020* and *Executive Summary.* The caregivers of special needs adults number is from the *2019*

C.A.R.E. Study. Caregiver age numbers are from Distribution of Informal Unpaid Caregivers Between 2015 and 2017 by age, Statistica, https://www.statista.com/statistics/1109910/share-of-informal-unpaid-caregivers-in-the-us-by-age.

11 "2023 Alzheimer's Disease Facts and Figures," Alzheimer's Association (2023).

12 Matthew Henry, *Matthew Henry's Commentary on the Whole Bible* (Peabody, MA: Hendrickson Publishers, 2008), 1376.

13 *Long-Term Caregiving: The True Costs of Caring for Aging Adults*, The Associated Press-NORC Center for Public Affairs Research; October 2018.

14 *2019 C.A.R.E. Study.*

15 *2019 C.A.R.E. Study.*

16 *Caregiving in the United States 2020.*

17 Caregiver Statistics: Demographics, Family Caregiver Alliance, https://www.caregiver.org/resource/caregiver-statistics-demographics/

18 *2019 C.A.R.E. Study.*

19 Edward G. Shaw, *The Dementia Care-Partner's Workbook: A Guide for Understanding, Education, and Hope* (Companion Press, 2019), 172.

20 *The Dementia Care-Partner's Workbook.*

21 Kymberly Grosso, "Do Couples Divorce Because of Autism?" March 3, 2011. *Psychology Today.* https://www.psychologytoday.com/intl/blog/autism-in-real-life/201103/do-couples-divorce-because-autism.

About the Author

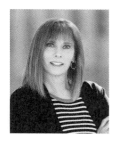 Debbie Barr is an author, health educator, and speaker with a passion for encouraging people to engage deeply with God as they journey through tough times.

She earned her bachelor's degree in journalism from the Pennsylvania State University and her master's degree in health education from East Carolina University. A master certified health education specialist (MCHES®), Debbie is especially interested in health and wellness, health literacy, and Christian growth.

She lives in Bermuda Run, North Carolina.

You can learn more about Debbie by visiting her website (debbiebarr.com), her Amazon author page (amazon.com/author/debbiebarr) or her Linkedin profile (www.linkedin.com/in/debbiebarr).

Hope and Healing

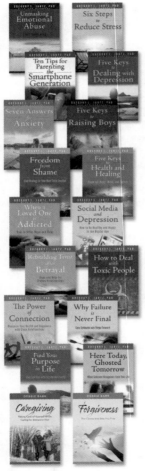

www.hendricksonrose.com